TABLE OF CONTENTS

A Necessary Disclaimer ▲

For legal reasons based on the prevailing societal paradigm, I include the following:

manifesto - *n. a public declaration of the beliefs, objectives and/or wisdom of an individual or entity.*

The purpose of this manifesto is to provide my *personal* experiences and observations about my health for anyone who wants to learn about these experiences. I am not a doctor—as that word is commonly used—and I do not claim to be one.

This information is not intended to be a substitute for professional advice from a "health professional." You should not use this information to diagnose or treat health issues or disease without consulting a qualified "health care provider" with any questions or concerns you may have regarding *your* condition, or ways in which to use alternative therapies. I, the author of this book, disclaim any personal liability or loss caused or alleged to be caused, through application of the information contained herein.

"In a world based on lies,
the truth is considered subversive"

1. Nature is Perfect ▲

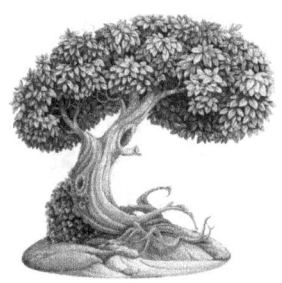

Here's a question for you: *"Do you believe nature is perfect or do you believe it is flawed?"* Do you believe there's an underlying intelligence and order to the way of natural things, or do you believe—in matters of health—that it's all random, a crap shoot of unpredictability, of chaos and luck, and that an imperfect nature requires mankind's help to improve upon it? What do you *really* believe?

Based on our behavior as a society, it is obvious most of us believe nature is actually flawed, hasn't quite gotten things right, and that our little blue pills, chemicals and drugs are what's needed to fix it.

I suggest to you that in order to take full advantage of the powerful healing forces I'm going to share with you, you must *start* with a belief that Nature is perfect.

Now, I'm not saying that nature is in a perfect state

at present. I'm saying that the principles, rules and laws that dictate how things operate were exquisitely and perfectly designed and continue to reflect that perfection...despite mankind's best efforts. Yes, there is pollution, there is climate change, oxygen depletion, and mass species extinctions that mankind has brought to the equation, but, despite this, there still remains something powerful upon which we can always rely.

Notice that I said it *starts* with your *belief* in, not with the *proof* of nature's perfection. The proof, if you require such, will actually come later—from your own experience.

A belief in nature's perfection is the cornerstone upon which the information in this manifesto is built. If you believe that nature is flawed, and that mankind is actually capable of improving upon it, then little else in this philosophy will make sense to you.

If you start with the premise that nature is perfect, life becomes a lot easier and certain choices and decisions become easier. If you start with the foundational belief that nature *is* perfect, it doesn't matter how many times the six o'clock news reports that GMOs are deemed safe by the Food & Drug Administration, you'll know there's no possible way man can improve upon nature. Period. You'll know that no canned vegetable can ever be better for you than one straight from the soil. You'll know there is no pharmaceutical that can ever really cure an illness.

From this belief system, you live beyond debate, beyond advertising, beyond marketing, beyond distraction, beyond the confusion that paralyzes others. You'll know that no drug can restore health; that no little blue pill can really restore vitality. Yes, they may mask symptoms, provide temporary relief, or force a temporary physical response, but there will *always* be side-effects because they are not natural. Period.

Now, here's the good news: there *are*, in fact, ways to get your hair to grow back, to restore the suppleness of your skin, to eliminate wrinkles, to restore your libido and vitality, to reverse the signs of aging and even cure cancer. However, those ways do not come from laboratory-made chemicals and pharmaceuticals. Those goals can be achieved through lifestyle changes, changes in diet, the use of herbs, foods, vitamins and minerals. I suggest to you that because nature is perfect, that these goals can be achieved through the use of sunlight, water, earth, air and time! It can be done through S.W.E.A.T. *(Pronounced just like its perspiration namesake!)* And once you know the secret to activating these natural forces to achieve and maintain your health, your life may never be the same!

2. The body is coded to heal ▲

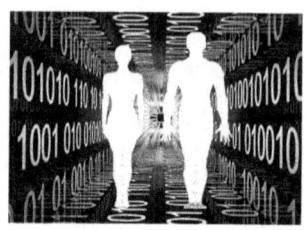

Now, because nature is perfect, your body, as part of that perfection, is *coded to heal.*

You already know this to be true. Ever since childhood, you've seen cuts and scrapes heal on their own. Bones mend. Headaches and other pains pass after a good night's sleep. You are always healing.

In fact, many conditions and feelings we think of as "illness" are actually the body's attempts to heal itself. Diarrhea is the body flushing foreign substances from the stomach and intestinal tract. The high temperature of a fever allows the body's immune system to function better and may kill bacteria and viruses that are sensitive to changes in temperature. Even the medical establishment refers to certain conditions as "self-limiting," meaning that—left to its own devices —the body will, in fact, limit and control these conditions without any interference from doctors.

And the best part is: you don't need experience or training to benefit from the coding. But it goes further!

The truth is, medicines don't heal the body. Always remember this. *In every case of true and lasting healing, it is the body's immune system that actually does the healing.* The purpose of real health care, therefore, should be to help the body heal itself. We'll be returning to this truth throughout this manifesto.

Now, not only will your body always endeavor to heal itself, it will heal its organs and internal systems in the appropriate sequence to optimize your body's resources for survival. In other words, if, for instance, you embark on a new nutrition campaign after years of deprivation, your body might have already shut down certain systems to conserve resources—perhaps you lost your hair, or your libido, or maybe your fingernails stopped growing. However, once you provide the body with proper nutrition, it will revive and reactivate those "deactivated" systems in the appropriate order. Your body innately knows how to allocate resources, and when to restore these organs and systems to optimize your chances of survival.

The important takeaway from this section is simply that there are innate mechanisms coded deep within your DNA that almost guarantee that, under the right conditions, your body will always return itself to normalcy. Those "right conditions" come from the use of sunlight, water, earth, air and time.

3. You are Your Own Authority ▲

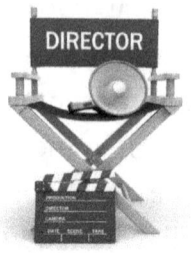

Now, *because* nature is perfect, and *because* the human body is inherently coded to heal, that means you—yes, you—are your own authority! In other words, thanks to nature, the mechanisms are already in place for you to achieve perfect health, long life and the fountain of youth. You don't need medical degrees or higher education in order to feel confident about making decisions about your body. The decision-making authority for how to care for your body rests within you, and you can do so confidently, provided you make those decisions within the right paradigm.

You—not the FDA, not doctors, not pharmacists, not the government, not the evening news anchors, not newspaper columnists, not the multitude of "theys" touting "the latest research" and studies—know more than you (in partnership with nature) about what's good or bad for you nor how to achieve true health.

If the prospect of being your own authority scares you, it's because we've all been led to believe that health is so complicated that one needs a degree in order to make even the most basic decisions.

Now, don't get me wrong. The modern medical care establishment serves a purpose. Your doctor may have seen certain conditions enough times to advise you in many ways. Tests and equipment exist to help diagnose symptoms. You *do* need training to know how to administer emergency care, CPR (Cardio-pulmonary resuscitation), or reset a broken bone correctly. However, nature has made the care and feeding of its handiwork foolproof enough that even the least among us can be successful at it, provided we follow some glaringly obvious guidelines.

The body may be complex in its operation, but the basic *knowledge* required for keeping it that way may be simpler than you think. For just as you don't need to be an electrician to flip on a light switch to get electricity to work for you; and just as pilots don't need to be jet engine mechanics to fly a plane, you too, with just some basic training, can be the director in charge of how your health journey proceeds.

And, yes,we're going to keep it simple.

4. There is Only One Illness ▲

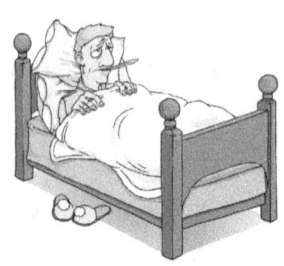

At this point, you may be thinking: *"Okay, even if I accept that nature is perfect and that the body is coded to heal, why am I and everyone I know always getting sick? Why aren't we healthy and rejuvenating instead of ill and deteriorating? Why do I have cancer, fibromyalgia, allergies or [fill in the blank]?"*

Great questions! The first thing to know is: it doesn't matter what *name* the medical establishment gives to a particular condition. While it's true that naming a set of symptoms can be helpful and ultimately lead to an appropriate course of treatment, most progressive healers agree there is only one real "illness." And that is...

Imbalance.

Think about this. If the root cause of a set of symptoms is that your body is out of balance, and you simply treat that set of symptoms (to which you've given a fancy name) without addressing the *cause* of the underlying imbalance, then that imbalance may show itself later as a completely new set of symptoms in a completely different part of the body. And that is precisely the fatal flaw with the approach that modern medicine often takes to what it calls health care, and why it all seems so complicated to most people. They focus on the multiplicity of *manifestations* of imbalance, while ignoring the underlying causes.

Yes, some people are born with weak hearts or lungs. I suggest, however—congenital defects aside—that whatever currently ails you is probably *not* something you were born with, but something that developed gradually over time, not because health is random and you're unlucky, and not because it's *"normal for someone your age."* It's most likely some dietary choice and/or lifestyle behavior or environmental exposure that's at the root of your health challenges. And the reason it won't go away on its own—and may even be getting worse—is not because nature isn't perfect, and not because the body isn't coded to heal, but because you keep doing the same thing and exposing yourself to the same environment every day while expecting different results! (I'm sure you've heard that concept before!)

Now, here's the simple secret: Imbalance is caused by either an accumulation or a deficiency, or both. In other words, *there's something inside the body that shouldn't be there, and/or there's something that <u>should</u> be inside the body that isn't.*

With this simple concept of illness as your guide, you'll find that making decisions and choices becomes simpler because—as you might correctly assume—if the *cause* of a condition can be expressed in simple terms, then the *solution* can be simply stated as well.

Understanding and maintaining health in nature's foolproof universe is simple. However, the more you deviate from what's natural, the more challenging and complicated it can become. Let's understand the strategy of maintaining health and effecting cure by understanding an equally simple formula.

5. Vitality is a formula ▲

$$\sigma = \sqrt{\frac{1}{N}\sum_{i=1}^{N}\left(x_i - \bar{x}\right)}$$
$$x = \frac{-b \pm \sqrt{b^2 - 4ac}}{2a}$$

Now, even though nature *is* perfect, and even though the body *is* coded to heal, and even as your own authority with a simplified concept of illness as your guide, you are not free to abuse your body or do anything you wish.

On the contrary, those truths are the very reasons why you, more than most and more than before, must now follow certain rules; for a body born of nature, *must* adhere to nature's rules to survive and to thrive.

The challenge most of us in modern society face— the issue that is at the root of our health challenges—is that we are attempting—whether knowingly or unknowingly—to maintain natural health in an unnatural environment and under unnatural conditions.

In other words, we are asking *"How can I get this body to maintain its natural operation even though I am forcing it to do unnatural things? How can I achieve optimal operation from a naturally-designed machine using alien input? How can I eat fast food, drink alcohol, smoke, sleep irregularly or not at all, breathe polluted air and take drugs, AND, at the same time, get this body to function as designed?"*

Furthermore, while attempting this nearly impossible feat, we are seeking health advice (a) from people who don't believe in nature's perfection or the simplicity of cure, (b) from institutions motivated solely by financial gain by selling us unnatural foods and unnatural cures, and (c) within a paradigm of treatment based on a compartmentalized rather than holistic approach to the human body.

Here's all you need to know to have the best overall understanding of the body and its operation: If you wish to remain vital, vibrant and virile, there is a simple formula. **The formula for vitality is:**

$$V = P^2 - O$$

V is VITALITY.

P^2 is POTENTIAL POWER: the available strength to keep you alive, drive the human machinery, and provide strength and endurance. You get this from the food you eat and its interaction with your body.

O is OBSTRUCTION: foreign matter, heavy metals, chemicals plaque, mucus, bacteria, viruses, parasites; anything hindering circulation, organ function and flow. In other words, blockage or toxicity.

In words, the formula is stated:

"Vitality equals Potential Power minus Obstruction"

To illustrate, let's say you have 100 of some imaginary units of potential power (P^2) in your body, but you have 25 units of obstruction (O) in your colon. The amount of vitality (V) that your body has available to expend, therefore, is only 75.

100(P^2)ower – 25(O)bstruction = 75(V)itality

You can see that as soon as the amount of "O" (obstruction) in your system becomes greater and greater and approaches the amount of "P" (potential power) the human machine must come to a standstill. For if you have 100 units of potential power, but have 99.999 units of obstruction, then your vitality is effectively ZERO, and you stop functioning. Yes, V = P^2 - O is the formula of life and of vitality, and at the same time you may call it the formula for illness and death as "O" becomes greater and greater.

At this point, you may be thinking: *"So, how do I increase my potential power, and decrease obstruction?"*

The answers are simple: 1. Eat real food. 2. Keep the body's cells clean.

6. A Definition of Real Food ▲

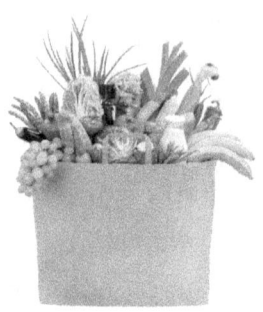

Understand this: Just because something can be chewed and swallowed does not make it real food!

The Ageless Adept's philosophy defines real food as *"unmodified, raw, enzyme-rich nuts, seeds, fruits and vegetables eaten in as close to their natural state as possible."* Boiled carrots, or carrots from a can are not the same as raw carrots. One is dead, one is alive. If you can't put it in the ground and grow another one, then, generally speaking, it's not real food. Period.

Furthermore, anything you do to food to take it out of its natural state, renders it less food. You dehydrate food and it's less food. You boil food and it's less food.

Hopefully, there'll come a time when you see the average western supermarket for what it is: a repository of ostensibly edible products created for the sole purpose of making a sale; cans, boxes and plastic containers of altered, boiled, cured, dyed, denatured, engineered, fried, frozen, flavored, filtered, hulled, injected, modified, pasteurized, preserved, supplemented and tainted objects that pass for food simply because they can be chewed and swallowed. You can do better.

Given the state of the various food-producing industries and industrial farming practices of planting genetically-modified seeds in nutrient-poor soil, spraying with pesticides and harvesting them before they are sufficiently ripe, it's increasingly challenging to find real food short of growing it ourselves.

The S.W.E.A.T. life strategy understands this challenge and advocates choosing a "reasonable facsimile" in the absence of the real thing. You can make the most practical effort to eat real food by choosing organic produce, incorporating raw food, "vitalizing" meals with superfoods and natural supplements, and adding non-pharmaceutical vitamins into your diet. These are the best ways to give the body what it requires even in our modern society.

Now, beyond giving the body what it needs to function properly and activate its natural healing code, there's something else required. You've got to keep the body's cells clean. And that requires a bit more than simply taking showers and going to the toilet!

7. A Clean Cell Never Dies ▲

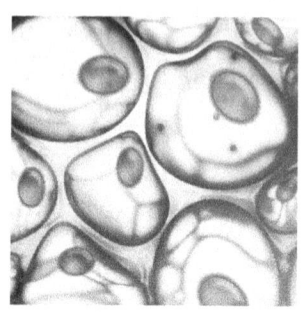

On January 17, 1912, Nobel Prize winner Dr. Alexis Carrel began a famous experiment at the Rockefeller Institute for Medical Research in which he placed tissue cultured from an embryonic chicken heart in a flask of his own design. He maintained the living culture for well over twenty years—much longer than a chicken's normal life span—proving that living cells could be kept alive indefinitely by simply controlling the nutrients and removing the waste in the surrounding solution.

Proper nutrition and removal of waste. This is the simple formula for longevity for which no practical lifestyle guide has ever existed. Our failure practicing this formula is the cause of most, if not all, disease.

--from the book, *A Clean Cell Never Dies*

While most of us are taught early in life how to cleanse externally and scrub our skin, wash our hair and brush our teeth, we are rarely taught to do an *internal* cleanse and cleanse the blood, scrub the colon, wash the liver, purge the kidneys or clean the lymphatic system as part of any regular maintenance.

The S.W.E.A.T. life strategy suggests colonics, coffee enemas, herb detoxes, saunas and other herbal as well as mechanical strategies to help push, pull or otherwise clean and expel toxins from the body's organs (with emphasis on the colon), systems, muscles and deep within tissues in order to achieve a state of internal cleanliness that can help the body remain youthful and vibrant.

Review

To review, there are seven critical concepts that form the basis of understanding and using the S.W.E.A.T. philosophy and protocol.

1. Nature is Perfect
2. The Body is Coded to Heal
3. You Are Your Own Authority
4. There is Only One Illness
5. Vitality is a Formula
6. There IS a Definition of Real Food
7. A Clean Cell Never Dies

To summarize: If you start with the premise that only nature—not man—can offer the human body its most appropriate, most effective, and only sustainable paradigm of **perfect** health, AND defer to your body's innate and **coded** wisdom to heal itself without pharmaceutical intervention, AND use your **authority** to make health decisions and lifestyle choices based not on advertising campaigns but on a basic understanding of the **one** cause of illness and the simplicity of cure, AND incorporate the **formula** for vitality and health into your daily life, AND commit to eating **real food** AND to keeping the body's cells **clean**, you will have the necessary mindset to get the most from the S.W.E.A.T. philosophy and protocol.

All that's needed now are the actual methods!

S.W.E.A.T ▲

"Ah, to live a life fantastic
and of vital health sublime
one need only harness sunlight,
water, earth, the air and time"

The Theory

The S.W.E.A.T. Manifesto contends that your body is best served and will achieve the most success in its efforts to survive and thrive if you incorporate *sunlight, water, earth, air and time* into its operation. This is what I call the S.W.E.A.T. life strategy.

Said with more detail: to the degree that you are able to expose your skin to direct sunshine, drink pure water, utilize and experience the unmodified feel, fauna and fruits of the earth, breathe oxygen-rich air and harness the power of the passage of time into your day-to-day existence as well as your efforts to heal, to that extent shall you achieve perfect health, long life and the fountain of youth. This strategy works because your body is coded to heal, your immune system is what actually does all true healing, and by following this life strategy you give your immune system its best tools for accomplishing its coded function.

The Unreasonable Expectation?

The challenge, of course, is how can we live this S.W.E.A.T. paradigm given the demands on our time and the dietary decisions that arise as a consequence of the career and lifestyle choices we often feel forced to make just to survive in a modern, capitalist age?

In other words, *"How can I live hang out in the sun when I have to rise at 6:00am to go to work for eight hours a day and don't return home until dark? How can I drink pure water when everything is either from a tap or from a bottle? How can I touch the earth when I live in a concrete jungle? How can I breathe oxygen-rich air when the city I must reside in to earn a living is polluted? How can I harness the power of the passage of time when my days are so filled?"*

The Reasonable Facsimile Solution

There is no easy solution. If it *were* easy, everybody would be doing it. It's going to require some courage and some discipline. Fortunately, however, there are ways to obtain the benefits of S.W.E.A.T. even within the constraints of a modern existence. This section offers an introduction to these *"reasonable facsimiles."* I invite you to research and explore them in more detail on your own or in the individual books in my Ageless Adept's series. [See "Books in the Series"]

8. Sunlight ▲

"If you lived life in the clime for which your body was designed..." you would spend more time in sunlight.

The sun's ultraviolet rays are antiseptic and can kill bacteria, viruses, fungi, yeasts, molds and mites in air and water, as well as on surfaces including the skin. Sunlight converts cholesterol in the skin to Vitamin D, and regulates bodily processes. The sun's infrared rays improve neuralgia, neuritis, arthritis and sinusitis. Sunlight regulates bodily processes, stimulates the pineal gland, and normalizes heart rate, blood pressure and respiration. It increases oxygen to the blood and thus improves muscular endurance.

Additionally, being in the sun means you would sweat more, which regulates body temperature, eliminates germs and bacteria, cleans the pores and releases toxins through the skin improving complexion. Sweating boosts immunity, improves mood, reduces hot flashes, releases growth hormones for faster healing, and releases pheromones that boost sexual arousal in others!

Instead of experiencing such exposure and benefits, we wear clothes almost entirely blocking the sun's rays, we lather on cancer-causing sunblock creams, use alzheimer-inducing and cancer-causing antiperspirants, drive in vehicles with tinted windows, and live and work in air-conditioned environments and never get to sweat.

Deficiency or insufficiency of natural sunlight and vitamin D has been associated with: adrenal insufficiency, Alzheimer's, allergies, autoimmune disorders including multiple sclerosis and rheumatoid arthritis, cancers of the colon, breast, skin and prostate, depression, seasonal affective disorder, diabetes 1&2, gluten intolerance, heart disease, hypertension, Metabolic Syndrome, infertility, sexual dysfunction, learning/behavior disorders, misaligned teeth, cavities, obesity, osteopenia, osteoporosis, rickets, Parkinsons, PMS and psoriasis.

Yes, the sun is the source of all life on the planet, yet many of us live in mortal fear of it and actively avoid it at every turn. To live the S.W.E.A.T. life strategy, that must change!

How to harness the power of sunlight

There's no substitute for real, *direct* sunlight (i.e. nothing between you and the sun except air; glass blocks the sun's infrared rays). Don't let "conventional wisdom" scare you away from soaking in the sun! Soak for at least one hour each day (shorter duration for people with paler, melanin-poor skin).

Reasonable Facsimiles

The s*unlight* in s*unlight-water-earth-air-time* also includes replicating the effects that exposure to sunlight would create, including sweating. Therefore, infrared saunas, dry saunas, vitamin D supplementation, as well as physical activity (and stopping the use of antiperspirants) to encourage sweating are all included in what I refer to as the "reasonable facsimiles" of sunlight!

Continue this journey in *The Sun Cure.*

***

Now, with more time spent in the sun, guess what? You'd probably feel like drinking more water, which— coincidentally or by nature's perfect design? You decide—is next in the S.W.E.A.T. life style requirements!

9. Water ▲

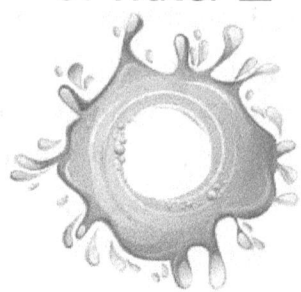

"If things were as pristine as in the world's creation scene...," you would be drinking cleaner water, with higher mineral content, higher levels of oxygen, without chlorine, without fluoride...and you'd probably drink more of it since it would taste so good!

With more water, the brain (which is 73% water) and its functions improve. Your cells would be hydrated and oxygenated, digestion, metabolism and flexibility would improve, your body would cleanse itself more regularly, and energy levels would increase! Drinking more water improves kidney function and reduces kidney stone formation, osteoporosis, hip fractures and heart disease.

Dr. F. Batmanghelidiji, author of *Your Body's Many Cries for Water*, writes, "I have seen water completely reverse conditions such as: asthma; angina; hypertension; migraine headaches; arthritis pain; back pain; colitis pain and chronic constipation; heartburn and hiatal hernia; depression; chronic fatigue syndrome; high cholesterol; morning sickness; overweight—even heart problems thought to need bypass surgery. All...have responded simply and permanently to water. Ordinary 'natural' water."

Dehydration causes fatigue, reduces overall motivation and endurance, affects mood, reduces cognitive function and motor skills, impairs memory, leads to dry skin and wrinkles and constipation, and is a cause of headaches, back pain and even bad breath!

How to harness the power of water

Drinking purified, fluoride-free, chlorine free, room temperature rain water would be best. Spring water is good. Reverse-osmosis and filtered water is good. (The best advice, despite what the officials say, is to stay away from tap water from municipal sources.) Fill a container with half-gallon to one gallon each day and drink throughout the day to stay hydrated.

Reasonable facsimiles

The *water* in s*unlight-water-earth-air-time* includes replicating water's effects both internally and externally. This includes various forms of hydrotherapy, colonics, enemas and drinking and bathing in ozonated and oxygenated water.

10. EARTH ▲

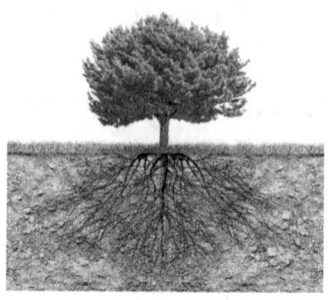

"*If your contact with the earth had been started right at your birth...,*" you would have had more direct physical contact with the soil and benefit from the earth's magnetic field and be more grounded in reality. You would have more knowledge of and faith in the life-sustaining benefits of plant life, herbs, fruits, vegetables, nuts and seeds, you would eat food that was closer to its natural raw state, organic, nutrient rich, and endowed with soil-borne organisms that would keep your intestinal tract healthy, you would experience the cleansing benefits of clay on your skin as well as inside your colon.

However, in our modern world, and particularly in what Reggae singer, Bob Marley, called the "concrete jungle," it is possible for someone to be born, live and die without their feet ever touching the actual soil of the earth. Think about it. A baby is born in a sanitized, concrete hospital. She's carried home in a metal car that touches asphalt. She lives her life in a high-rise apartment, and walks to school in shoes on cement sidewalks. During her working life, she travels to the office in steel trains. She lives her most of her entire life—every waking and sleeping moment—separated from the earth hundreds of feet above the ground. And if, on that infrequent occasion she seeks natural settings free of concrete or asphalt—hopefully, she may go to the beach on occasion and walk barefoot on the sand, or go to a park—there's a good chance she may wear sandals that still separate her from the actual living earth. And, to take a few steps back in time, remember, she was conceived and began the very instant of life in the womb of a woman who, herself, may never have touched the grounding and rejuvenating effect of actually connecting to the earth.

What effect do you think that might have on the world view, thought processes, bodily functions, and even basic humanity of an individual, family or society that never touches ground—people who are never, you might say, "grounded?"

In electrical terms, to "ground" an object means just that, to connect it to the earth. When an electrical appliance operates, it will build up an electrical charge. The earth naturally attracts excess electrical charge and dissipates it so that it does not accumulate and cause harm to the user. You ground something to keep it functioning properly and so it doesn't cause harm to itself or to others. Walking on the soil allows your body to absorb negative electrons which balances the positive charge we accumulate from the magnetic fields of electrical appliances, power lines, cell phones/towers and x-ray scanners are all around us.

How to harness the power of earth

You should make it a point to walk barefoot directly upon the earth and clay—not a concrete sidewalk or an elevated park. Walking on the beach, touching and even sleeping on the earth and eating clay all keep you "grounded."

Reasonable Forms & Facsimiles

The *earth* in *sunlight-water-earth-air-time* also includes replicating earth's effects both internally and externally, both chemically and mechanically. This includes eating bentonite (and other types of) clay, diatomaceous earth and Himalayan pink salt in addition to clay baths (which have been shown to help children with autism) and magnetic therapy.

Additionally, *earth* includes the "fauna and fruits" of the earth. In other words, herbs, plants, vegetables and fruits in as close to their natural state as possible.

11. AIR ▲

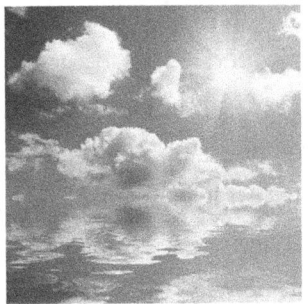

If each breath that you took in gave you enough pure oxygen, your entire body would function better. Anaerobic bacteria would not survive in your system.

You can go without water for a few days. You can do without sunlight, you can do without food for many days. Without air, you die in minutes. Therefore, air is arguably the most important element when looking to heal a specific condition, rejuvenate and grow younger. It is believed there was a time when the oxygen content in air was as high as 50%. Now it's less than 20% and even lower in major cities. The more you can do to introduce oxygen into the system, the more optimally the body will function.

Increasing the amount of oxygen in the body, whether through the facsimiles below, or often simply by deep breathing exercises can improve brain and nerve function, eyesight and hearing, kill bacteria and heal infections, reduce chronic pain and depression, cure ulcers and speed wound healing and recovery time from burns and strokes. In fact, so many of our ills are caused by bacteria and parasites that thrive in low-oxygen environments (anaerobic), that the list of ills that can be eased by increasing oxygen, say by hydrogen peroxide includes Allergies, Alzheimer's, Anemia, Arrhythmia, Asthma, Bronchitis, Cancer, Candida, Cardiovascular Disease, Cerebral Vascular Disease, Chronic Pain, Diabetes Type 11, Diabetic Gangrene, Diabetic Retinopathy Epstein-Barr Infection, Emphysema, Food Allergies, Fungal Infections, Gingivitis, Herpes Simplex/Zoster, HIV, Influenza, Liver Cirrhosis, Lupus Erythematosis, Multiple Sclerosis, Parasitic Infections, Parkinsonism, Periodontal Disease, Prostatitis, Rheumatoid Arthritis, Shingles, Sinusitis, Sore Throat, Ulcers, Viral Infections, Warts, and Yeast Infections.

Reasonable Forms & Facsimiles

The *air* in s*unlight-water-earth-air-time i*ncludes getting oxygen to the cells through H2O2 (Hydrogen Peroxide), DMSO, Ozone therapy, MMS (orally; hot bath; enemas). It also includes exposing the body and skin to air. See *The Sun Cure* for a discussion.

12. t I m e ▲

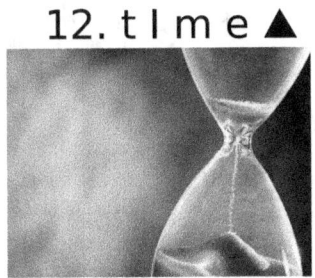

"And if your paradigm of cure, could let you wait more and endure...," you might enjoy degrees of healing and rejuvenation that would astound you!

So, how do you invoke the passage of time to cure your illness?

Fasting.

An extended water fast—going several days without solid food and drinking only water—allows the body the time to stop, rest, shift gears and direct the energy it would normally use for *digestion* towards *healing*. Remember, in all situations, regardless of the protocol, it is your immune system that does the healing and it always follows nature's timetable.

If you could "endure" the healing crises and retracings (healing illnesses in reverse order to their first occurrence) that happen during a fast—beginning from Stage 1 (Days 1 to 2), to Stage 2 (Days 3 to 7), to Stage 3 (Days 8 to 15), to Stage 4 of your fast (Days

16 to 30) and beyond—you might just find that the colon is repaired, acidic blood chemistry is corrected, old injuries are permanently healed, tumors are metabolized, scar tissue and arthritic deposits dissolve; damaged organs regain lost function, the lymphatic system is thoroughly cleaned and mental clarity, emotional balance, memory and concentration improve dramatically! *(I can attest to these last few Stage 4 benefits having recently fasted for 17 days!)*

Unfortunately, there is no substitute or *reasonable facsimile* for the passage of time. You must simply resolve, commit, find the courage and discipline, then just do it! Here's a final suggestion, however, to help with that resolve: When it comes to your current state of health, instead of focusing on what you can and can't eat, and lamenting what foods aggravate this or that condition, choose to "reboot" your body (which is what a fast does), it just might "reset" your digestive system to how it was *before* those sensitivities developed, and you might find you can eat just about anything...just like you did in times past!

Intrigued? Continue this journey harnessing the power of time in the book, *Fast & Grow Young!*

In closing, enjoy the following poetic encapsulation of the ideas behind the S.W.E.A.T. life practices:

sublime ▲

sublime – *adj*. of such excellence, grandeur, or beauty as to inspire great admiration or awe. *Synonyms: exalted, elevated, noble, lofty, awe-inspiring, awesome, majestic, magnificent, imposing, glorious, supreme!*

If you lived life in the clime
for which your body was designed

And if things were as pristine
as in the world's creation scene

And if your contact with the earth
had begun right at your birth

And if each breath that you took in
gave you enough pure oxygen,

And if your paradigm of cure,
would let you wait more and endure

Then you could live a life fantastic
and of vital health sublime
by simply harnessing the sunlight,
water, earth, the air and time!

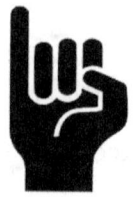

Manifesto CONCLUSION ▲

SWEAT—*sunlight, water, earth, air and time*—form the underlying basis of all true health and the essence of all real cure. This is my belief.

If you need to, you can look for and find new research and studies being published every day that confirm the truth and benefits of everything you've read in this manifesto...if you need to. Know, however, that these truths are only "new" or "amazing" in societies who, sadly, believe themselves superior to nature's perfection, and who put more faith in laboratory experiments than in the clearly obvious examples and foolproof operations manual that nature provides. You don't need studies to prove what's patently obvious.

However much faith or hope you may have in the efficacy of modern drugs; however much you may believe that health *insurance* is the best strategy for health *care*; however much you may believe that health is random or genetic; however much you may believe that we're all just "flying blind" and that this is all an experiment, my goal is to introduce those who believe to another set of beliefs, another set of choices and another set of possible outcomes.

What I've learned over the years is that if you do the work required to prove some of these beliefs, to make some of these choices and experience these outcomes, you just may find yourself in an entirely different world of possibilities.

I can make no guarantees. However, I *can* share with you a pledge I made to *myself*, a promise I've kept now for most of my life, that has kept me feeling youthful and endowed me with the wisdom to be able to help others in certain parts of this journey:

The S.W.E.A.T Manifesto Pledge ▲

"I will find the courage and discipline to eat only what exists in Nature, avoid unnatural substances and environments, bask daily in sunshine, maintain direct contact with the earth, breathe clean air, purge the colon, cleanse the system, fast when dis-eased, and live passionately and on purpose from a belief system of universal perfection. I will keep the cells of the body clean, prevent illness, reverse aging, rejuvenate the body, achieve perfect health and long life and become my own fountain of youth!"

BONUS: Are we all simply flying blind?

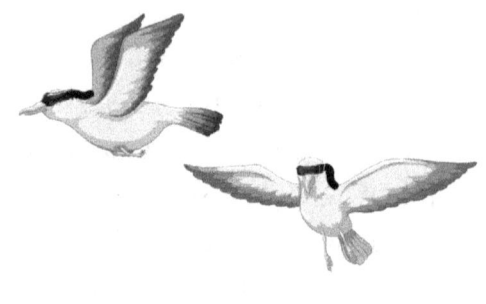

▲

After reading the *S.W.E.A.T Manifesto* and its emphasis on living a nature-guided lifestyle, you may be as excited as I (still) am about sharing this information with friends and family. Be warned, however, that in doing so, many "newbies" encounter resistance and even ridicule from friends, relatives and even strangers, and find themselves in heated arguments about the safety or sanity of such a lifestyle to individuals as well as to the planet. My best advice is never get into such arguments in the first place!

There's an old saying: *"A man convinced against his will is of the same opinion still."* In other words, you really shouldn't make it your mission to attempt to convince people of things they aren't willing to believe. (The resistance I encounter from friends and family, even today, after having published over a dozen books on the subject, is *my* greatest frustration.)

There is, however, something YOU can learn by

understanding some of the reasons people justify, defend, resist, ridicule and attack these ideas. It may help *you* remain steadfast in your own beliefs, so that *they* don't talk *you* out of them!

I've concluded that people resist because of the following beliefs—presented here along with what S.W.E.A.T. philosophy offers in response:

1. They believe this is all a cosmic experiment and that health is a random game of chance within a flawed universe. SWEAT SAYS: *Nature is Perfect.*

2. They believe that health comes from drugs or other forces outside of themselves. SWEAT SAYS: *The body is coded to heal.*

3. They are confused about whom to believe. SWEAT SAYS: *You are your own authority*

4. They believe illness and healing are complicated matters. SWEAT SAYS: *There is only one disease*

5. They believe that "more is better" and that constantly eating is the only key to survival and vitality. SWEAT SAYS: *Vitality has a formula*

6. They have an incorrect, inadequate or non-existent definition of "food" and will blindly trust anything available in a supermarket or served in a restaurant as

being approved and acceptable for consumption.
SWEAT SAYS: *There is a definition of "real food."*

7. They believe in the inevitability of certain types of deterioration due to the passage of time, and feel powerless to do anything about it. SWEAT SAYS: *A clean cell never dies.*

8. This one is key: You'll often hear people quote some version of *"My grandfather smoked cigars and ate pork and drank alcohol and [insert vice here] every day of his life and lived to be 98 years old!"*

(To that, I think to myself: There are also stories of people who fall out of ten-story buildings and survive. Does that mean jumping out of ten-story buildings is a good idea? Performer 50 Cent was shot nine times and survived. Does that mean we'll all have the same result if we get shot 9 times? Don't allow others to use one specific exception to invalidate the general rule!)

What they're really saying is *"No one really knows, do they?"* *"No one has the secret."* They believe, in other words, that we are all simply "flying blind."

The truth is, we *do* know! We know that cigarettes cause cancer, that MSG is poison, that cow's milk and high-acid protein diets cause osteoporosis, that meat production increases methane and contributes to global warming! We know, and the fact that the sale of these items continues has everything to do with capitalism (and is an indication that the FDA does *not* really have your best interests at heart) and nothing to do with any uncertainty about their safety or their effects on the human body or the planet.

People whose belief system holds that nature is flawed, that illness is complicated, that drugs and insurance are the answers to health care, that "experts" and the "latest research" must be smarter than they are, and that anything in a supermarket approved for sale by the relevant government agency and that is edible is actually safe for consumption, that deterioration is inevitable, and that we're all, in essence, simply flying blind, see no reason to change. Why would they? It explains why they justify, defend and resist (attack and ridicule may show a lack of tact on their part, but...). It explains in part they're choice to keep doing what they're doing. It makes complete sense.

However, arming yourself with the SWEAT belief system and any rebuttals it offers isn't about winning arguments. You can't "win" an argument with someone who is closed-minded about your lifestyle. This journey is about finding and acting upon truths to improve *your own* health. With that said, however, it's natural to want to share what you've discovered with those you care about. In that case, I suggest your best strategy may simply be to set a good example. People who observe that you walk the talk, that you look years younger than your calendar age, and that you glow with an inexplicable vitality might be inspired to ask what exactly you are doing.

During a recent visit to New York, I ran into my friend, Andy. I hadn't seen Andy in over ten years, and his first comment upon seeing me was *"Wow, you look exactly the same as last time I saw you!"* So, later that day, when we started talking about *his* health, and when I suggested he do an extended water fast as a way to heal and rejuvenate, he was much more open.

Read Andy's 10-day fast testimony: www.fastandgrowyoung.com

***

Years ago, when I was first becoming vegan, I read a great book entitled *Why Do Vegetarians Eat Like That,* by David Gabbe. It's out of print, but you might be able to find copies for sale on Amazon or eBay! It's written in a question and answer format with short, easy-to-remember answers and rebuttals to the common challenges people use to question, discredit and even ridicule the notion that a plant-based diet is an objectively better lifestyle choice; questions to justify maintaining their current lifestyle choices including: *"Where do you get your protein?" "Doesn't milk do a body good?" "They say eggs are good for you?" "My religion says it's okay to eat meat,"* plus a ton of other questions and beliefs answered with a balance of common sense as well as facts and figures! Great book! My point is that books like this have been written to address those sorts of conversations. On the other hand, a person who really wants to learn a new way of thinking and behaving will engage in entirely different conversations. *"Where do you shop?" "Can you recommend some recipes?" "Wow! You look great! Are you doing something different?" "Can you show me how to make Kimchee?"* Those are the conversation-starters of someone who is open to what you represent. Spend your time and energy there!

***

For your own sanity, you should accept the reality that people are free to believe anything they wish to believe. You are your own authority. You don't anyone's validation or permission to engage in this lifestyle. Nor do you need to convince anyone to change theirs. Again, the best strategy is to avoid such arguments altogether. Just because someone says something or asks you a question that challenges your lifestyle doesn't mean you have to get defensive and answer with facts, figures, charts, research, rebuttal or proof. Your life will be much easier if you simply learn to reply, *"Yep, you're absolutely right."*

Let's practice, shall we?

NOT YOU: *"All things in moderation, I always say."*
YOU: *"Yep, you're absolutely right!"*

NOT YOU: *"People have been eating meat since the caveman days!"*
YOU: *"Yep, you're absolutely right!"*

See how easy that is?

Remember, when it comes to certain truths regarding health, the individual's agreement is not required. In other words, you (as well as friends and family) can believe anything you wish, but believing a falsehood will not change objective reality. For example, you can believe that crossing the street with your eyes closed is okay because *"drivers ALWAYS stop for pedestrians,"* and that belief system may serve you for a while, but sooner or later, objective reality will catch up with you. You can choose to believe that drinking cow's *"milk does a body good,"* but that won't stop how it aggravates your allergies, or how the high acidic content weakens your bones.

So, while we all may indeed be "flying blind" when it comes to certain aspects of life in this plane of dimensional reality, there *are* some things we absolutely know for sure that are beyond debate despite the efforts of certain special interests to contrive debates to keep us mired in confusion, and despite people's choices to believe otherwise.

The *S.W.E.A.T. Manifesto* is but one step along a path to get beyond those debates, to escape the confusion and empower you to become your own authority in the quest for perfect health, long life, and the fountain of youth. I hope it has been helpful!

Walt F.J. Goodridge,
Ageless Adept

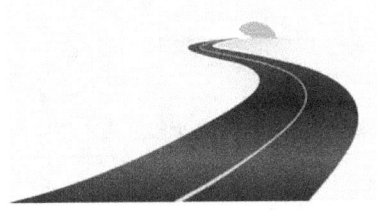

The Path ▲

"Perfect health, long life and eternal youth are not the random, genetic blessings of a chaotic or capricious universe, but natural birthrights that can be accessed through the mindful acceptance of simple truths, activated by the disciplined practice of proven activities, and sustained by advancement along a known path.
This is that path." --**The Ageless Adept**

a S.W.E.A.T. Life routine ▲
(a few of my own practices and their SWEAT connection
Download at www.sweatmanifesto.com)

MY S.W.E.A.T. LIFE MAINTENANCE ROUTINE

Daily Practice/Product	Sunlight	Water	Earth	Air	Time	Notes
▶ Solé *(Himalayan pink salt + water)*			✓			*Contains 84 minerals; 1tsp in morning*
▶ Oil Pulling			✓			*virgin coconut oil w/drop oil of oregano*
▶ Pushups	✓					
▶ Headstand/inversion						*10 min each morning*
▶ Barefoot run on the beach	✓		✓	✓		*3 miles every other day; shirtless*
▶ MSM			✓			
▶ Sunbath	✓			✓		*one hour each day; naked*
▶ H2O2 drops				✓		*6-10 drops every other day*
Weekly/Bi-weekly Practice/Product	**Sunlight**	**Water**	**Earth**	**Air**	**Time**	**Notes**
▶ Sauna	✓					*See instructions for detox sauna*
▶ 24-72 hour fast					✓	
▶ MMS* hot bath *(chlorine dioxide)*		✓		✓		*research Miracle Mineral Solution*
▶ Coffee enema			✓			
▶ H2O2 enema		✓		✓		*Use only Food grade H2O2*
6-Monthly/Annual Practice/Product	**Sunlight**	**Water**	**Earth**	**Air**	**Time**	**Notes**
▶ Extended water fast		✓		✓		*7 or more days*
▶ Colonic		✓				

The s.w.e.a.t. Infographic ▲
(Download FREE at www.sweatmanifesto.com)

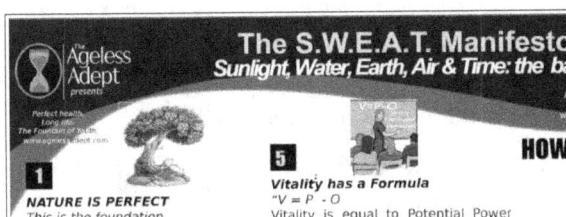

The S.W.E.A.T. Manifesto
Sunlight, Water, Earth, Air & Time: the basis of all cure

The Ageless Adept presents

Perfect health, Long life: The Foundation of Youth www.agelessadept.com

A free download from
The Ageless Adept
www.agelessadept.com
Print, post & share!

1

NATURE IS PERFECT
This is the foundation
An underlying intelligence governs how your body functions and doesn't require man to improve upon it. Nature is perfect, we are of nature, and real cure and health for natural beings can never come from lasers in labs or chemicals in capsules!

2

The Body Is Coded To Heal
And is always healing
Wounds heal, bones mend, colds pass, among a million other fixes the immune system does without intervention. It's our nature-endowed "healing code."

3

You Are Your Own Authority
..no degree needed!
You don't need a PhD to know that a carrot in a box can never be as beneficial as one straight from the soil. You don't need anyone's permission to eat an apple!

4

There Is Only One Illness
The single issue of imbalance—regardless of the name the doctors give it, is caused by either accumulation or deficiency. There's something in that should be out, or something out that should be in!

Take the Longevity Predictor Test
www.agelessadept.com/longevity-test

5

Vitality has a Formula
"$V = P - O$"
Vitality is equal to Potential Power minus Obstruction. The more toxicity, accumulation and obstruction, the less energy. Remove obstruction and experience increased vitality and health!

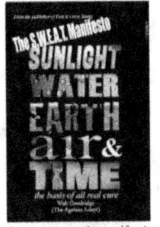

Order at www.sweatmanifesto.com

6

Real Food
Just because something can be chewed and swallowed doesn't make it real food. Real food is "unmodified, raw, enzyme-rich nuts, seeds, fruits or vegetables eaten in as close to their natural state as possible"

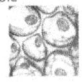

7

A Clean Cell Never Dies
Remember this truth, and you'll have one of the secrets to longevity. Live by it, and you may have the secret to immortality!

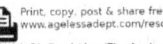

Print, copy, post & share freely! More
www.agelessadept.com/resources
©Walt F.J. Goodridge (The Ageless Adept)

HOW S.W.E.A.T. CURES

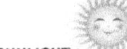

SUNLIGHT
Ultraviolet rays kill germs, spur Vitamin D production, boost immunity and improve mood. Get at least an hour each day...or a reasonable facsimile thereof to experience its effects.

WATER
Hydration improves brain, heart and kidney function, aids digestion, metabolism motor skills and flexibility, and improves complexion. Drink pure, living water!

EARTH
Ground yourself each day, eat or bathe in clay, experience the feel, fauna and fruit of the earth...or a reasonable facsimile thereof!

AIR
Oxygen kills bacteria and viruses, improves brain function, and increases energy. Supplement with oxygen therapies like food grade H_2O_2 and other reasonable facsimiles to reap the benefits.

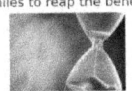

TIME
Fasting allows the body to rest so the immune system can purge, detox, heal and rejuvenate on nature's timetable. Read Fast & Grow Young for instructions at www.fastandgrowyoung.com

Website & Blog: www.agelessadept.com

Who is the Ageless Adept? ▲

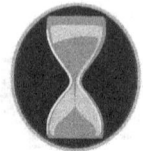

"Perfect health, long life and eternal youth are not the random, genetic blessings of a chaotic or capricious universe, but natural birthrights that can be accessed through the mindful acceptance of simple truths, activated by the disciplined practice of proven protocols, and sustained by advancement along a known path. This is that path."

My name is Walt F.J. Goodridge, author and publisher of the *Ageless Adept*™ series, and I'm here to prove a point!

Years ago, before I became vegan, a friend asked a question over lunch I couldn't answer. He asked, *"Do you know what's in the food you're eating?"* I did not, and it bothered me that I didn't, and so--with health, longevity and vitality as my goals--I dedicated my life to a search for answers and to *"share what I know, so that others may grow."*

My childhood in the Caribbean steeped in me an understanding of and reverence for our natural world of sunshine, water, earth, air and time. As an adult, I discovered that what passes as *normal* health and healing in the western paradigm is shockingly *unnatural*! It never made sense that we should need to turn to men in lab coats with pills in search of wellness. It makes more sense that Nature would have the answers built in; our bodies would have an innate healing code; our "operations manual" would be simple and foolproof.

Through my experiments, testimonials of others of like mind, and corroboration of researchers from this and previous eras, I've realized that the symptoms we as a society accept as a "normal" aging are the body's reactions to unnatural habits of ingesting pharmaceuticals, fake food with non-food ingredients, pesticides, hormones, steroids and antibiotics, as well as other environmental factors. Some of the habits may be hard to break, but are ultimately under our control. And, if the *causes* are controllable, then the *effects* are not inevitable and may even be reversible! That's what I'm here to prove!

I've distilled my results into a philosophy and information I hope will (1) empower you to become your own authority in health matters, and (2) make better survival choices from among the products and practices you'll encounter on your own path!

The Ageless Adept™ Series ▲

Free resources available exclusively at www.agelessadept.com/shop

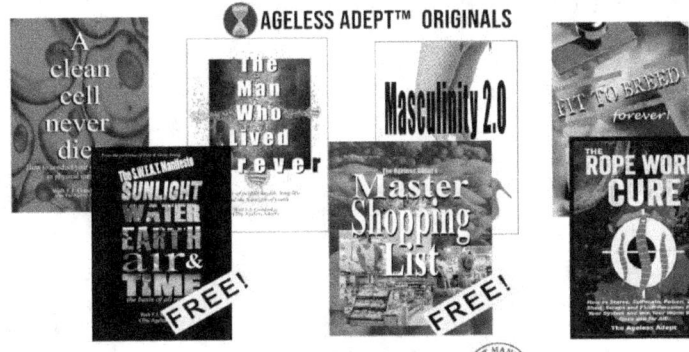

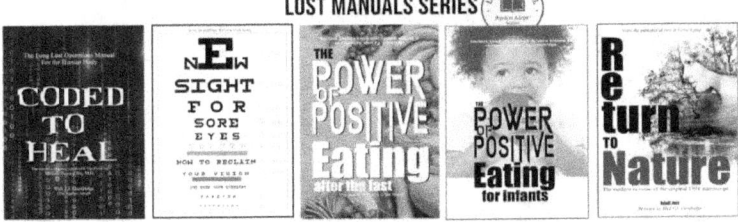

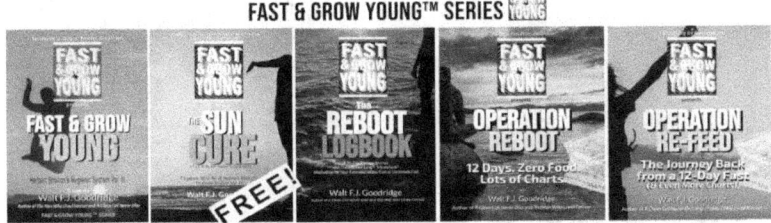

/see also: www.fastandgrowyoung.com

The Ageless Adept Resources ▲

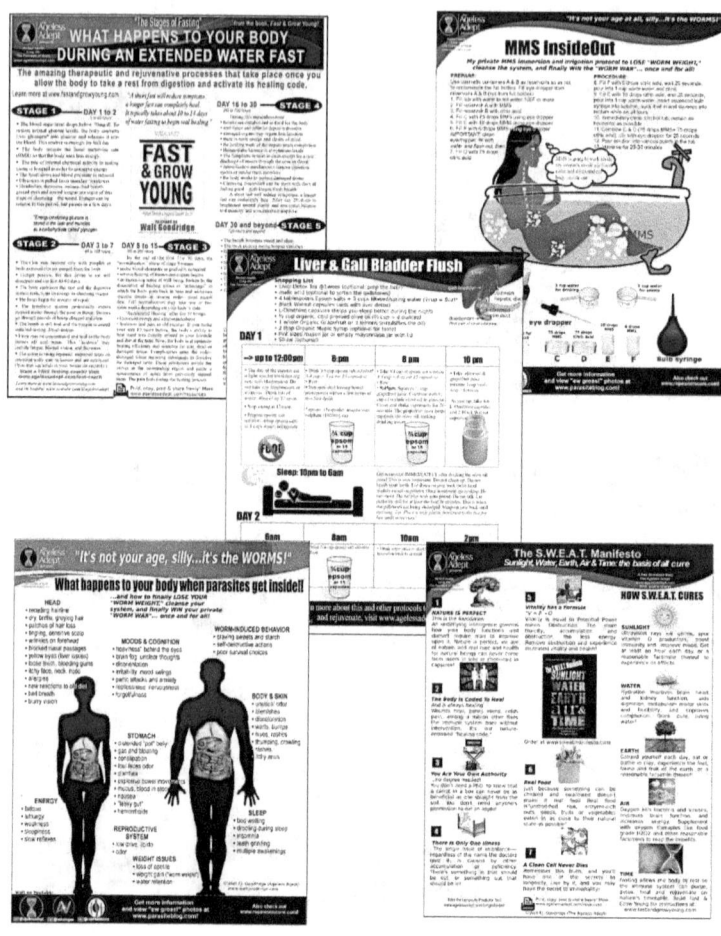

Free resources available exclusively at www.agelessadept.com

Watch, Read, Wear & Learn ▲

Youtube™ Channels

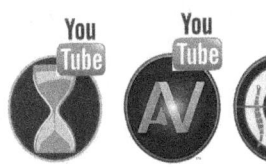

@agelessadept
@askavegan
@ropewormcure

Blogs

agelessadept.com/blog
parasiteblog.com

***

Merchandise

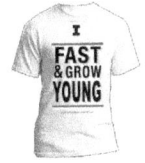 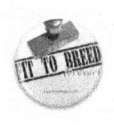

T-shirts, mugs, buttons and more!

Tests & Quizzes

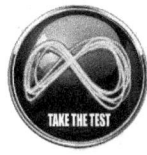 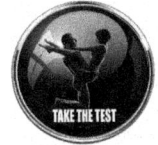

*Longevity Test
Fit to Breed? Test*

Available at www.agelessadept.com

Join the Ageless Adept Movement

"Get exclusive healing protocols, behind-the-scenes insight, and subscriber discounts on books & coaching."

https://www.agelessadept.com/newsletter

The Underlying Basis of all Real Cure

What if real healing doesn't come from a pill, procedure, or prescription?

What if the most powerful cures have no brand name, no expiration date, and no marketing department—because they've always been freely available in nature?

In this radical, compact guide, wellness advocate Walt F.J. Goodridge reclaims the original healing forces of the planet—Sunlight, Water, Earth, Air, and Time—as the only true foundation for lifelong health, resilience, and vitality.

Rejecting today's overcomplicated, pharmaceutical-driven approach to wellness, The S.W.E.A.T. Manifesto returns to first principles: the body is self-healing. Nature is the physician. Real cure is coded into your cells.

You'll explore the biological logic behind each of these five natural forces, discover why aging is not calendar-based but condition-based, and learn how to begin a practical return to balance—starting today.

Whether you're suffering from chronic fatigue, looking to extend your healthspan, or simply seeking truth in an industry full of conflicting advice, this book is your call to reawaken the healer within.

Because the truth is simple.

And a clean cell never dies.

Other Brands by the Author ▲

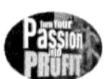 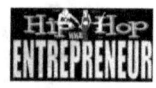 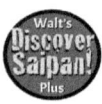

PassionProfit.com   JamaicaninAsia.com   HpHopEntrepreneur.com   DiscoverSaipan.com

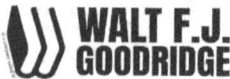

Or find them all at https://www.waltgoodridge.com